Nursing Mnemonics: 94 Memory Tricks to Demolish Nursing School

NRSNG.com | NursingStudentBooks.com

Jon Haws RN CCRN

©TazKai LLC 2015 and beyond

Reviews greatly help this book reach more students. Click below to leave a review on Amazon or to share the book on Facebook. Nothing helps more than a few kind words.

1

Contents

Obstetrics/ Pediatrics 12

Cyanotic Defects 12

Episiotomy- Evaluation of Healing 14

Fetal Accelerations and Decelerations 15

Fetal Well-Being- Assessment Tests 16

Intra Uterine Device- potential problems with use 17

PAINS 17

OB Non-Stress Test -3 negatives in a row to interpret results of Non-Stress Test 18

Oral Birth Control Pills- Serious Complications 19

Post-Partum Assessment 20

Severe Pre-Eclampsia- Signs and Symptoms 21

Hypoxia- Signs and Symptoms (in Pediatrics) 22

Child Abuse/Neglect- Warning Signs 23

Cleft Lip - Post Op Care 24

Tracheal Esophageal Fistula- Sign and Symptoms 26

Labs 27

Hyperkalemia- Causes..................................27

Hyperkalemia- Signs and Symptoms..................28

Hyperkalemia- Management..................30

Hypernatremia- Signs and Symptoms..................31

Hypernatremia- Signs and Symptoms..................32

Hypernatremia- Cause..................33

Hypernatremia- Management..................34

Hypocalcemia- Signs and Symptoms..................36

Hyponatremia- Signs and Symptoms..................37

Hyponatremia- Signs and Symptoms..................38

Electrolytes- Location in body..................39

Pharmacology..................40

Beta 1 and Beta 2..................40

Drugs for Bradycardia & Low Blood Pressure..................41

Drug Interactions..................42

Emergency Drugs..................43

Lidocaine Toxicity..................44

Steroid- Side Effects..................45

Mental Health..................46

Anorexia- Signs and Symptoms..................46

Bulimia- Signs and Symptoms 48

Bulimia- Signs and Symptoms 49

Alcoholism- Behavioral Problems 50

Alcoholism- Outcome 51

Depression Assessment 52

Manic Attack- Signs and Symptoms 53

Alzheimer- Diagnosis 54

Dementia 55

Senile Dementia- Assess for Changes 56

Med Surg 57

Med Surg 57

Arterial Blood Gases 57

Pulmonary Edema- Treatment 58

Dyspnea 59

Hypoxia- Signs and Symptoms 60

Asthma- Management 61

Diabetes Mellitus Type 1- Signs & Symptoms 64

Hyperglycemia/Hypoglycemia 65

Hypoglycemia- Signs and Symptoms 66

Circulatory Checks 67

Hypertension- Nursing Care..................................68

Hypertension- Complications...............................69

Heart Sounds...70

Cardiac Valves Blood Flow 71

Myocardial Infarction- Immediate Treatment.....72

Myocardial Infarction- Management....................74

Heart Failure- Right-Sided...................................75

Heart Failure- Left-Sided.....................................76

CHF- Treatment...77

Inflammation- Signs and Symptoms 79

Toxicty/Sepsis- Signs and Symptoms 81

Cancer- Early Warning Signs 82

Cancer- Interventions 83

Leukemia- Signs and Symptoms..........................84

Appendicitis- Assessment 85

    PAINS...85

Epiglottitis - Signs and Symptoms.......................86

Cholinergic Crisis...87

Adrenal Gland Hormones.....................................88

Cranial Nerve Mnemonic 01 89

Cranial Nerve Mnemonic 02 91

Cranial Nerve Mnemonic 03 92

Cranial Nerve Mnemonics- Sensory, Motor or Both..............93

Prostate 94

Diarrhea- treatment 95

Transient Incontinence- Common Causes 96

Transient Incontinence- Common Causes 96

Promotion and Evaluation of Normal Elimination.............97

Bleeding Precautions 98

Trauma- Complications 99

Trauma- Assessment (Emergency) 100

Trauma Surgery- After initial assessment.................102

Exercise Guidelines 103

Osteoporosis- Risk Factors.............................104

Dialysis- Who needs dialysis?...........................105

Gluten Free Diet..............................107

Nursing Fundamentals 108

Body Systems 108

Steps in the Nursing Process...........................110

Steps in the Nursing Process...........................111

Sprains and Strains- Nursing Care 112

Traction- Nursing Care 113

ADLs (Activity of Daily Living) 114

IADLS (Instrumental Activities of Daily Living) 115

Canes 116

Walkers 117

Disclaimer

Medicine and nursing are continuously changing practices. The author and publisher have reviewed all information in this book with resources believed to be reliable and accurate and have made every effort to provide information that is up to date with best practices at the time of publication. Despite our best efforts we cannot disregard the possibility of human error and continual changes in best practices the author, publisher, and any other party involved in the production of this work can warrant that the information contained herein is complete or fully accurate. The author, publisher, and all other parties involved in this work disclaim all responsibility from any errors contained within this work and from the results from the use of this information. Readers are encouraged to check all information in this book with institutional guidelines, other sources, and up to date information. For up to date disclaimer information please visit: http://www.nrsng.com/about.

Photo Credits:

All photos are original photos taken or created by the author or rights purchased at Fotolia.com. All rights to appear in this book have been secured.

Some images within this book are either royalty-free images, used under license from their respective copyright holders, or images that are in the public domain. Images used under a creative commons license

Your Free Gift!

As a way of saying thanks for your purchase, I'm offering a free PDF download:

"63 Must Know NCLEX® Labs"

With these charts you will be able to take the 63 most important labs with you anywhere you go!

You can download the 4 page PDF document by clicking here, or going to NRSNG.com/labs

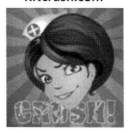
Introduction

Mnemonics and memory aids are one of the best ways for students to accelerate their learning.

This book contains 94 mnemonics specifically designed for nurses and nursing students preparing for the NCLEX® and who simply want to take their career to the next level.

The book is divided into sections based on nursing core content. With these mnemonics, colored pictures and detailed descriptions you will find yourself engaging and learning at a fast pace and retaining the information that you learn.

Be patient with yourself and take your time to learn the mnemonics that apply to the material you are currently learning or studying in school.

Learn more about our books at NursingStudentBooks.com or NRSNG.com. You can also contact me directly at contact@nrsng.com

Obstetrics/ Pediatrics

Cyanotic Defects

The 4 Ts

Tetralogy of Fallot
Truncus Arteriosus
Transposition of the Great Vessels
Tricuspid Atresia

Cyanotic heart defects are a group of congenital heart defects that result from deoxygenated blood by-passing the lungs and going into systemic circulation. Tetralogy of Fallot includes 4 anatomical abnormalities that are pictured below. Truncus Arteriosus is a condition where the pulmonary trunk and aorta don't properly divide in development. This results in one large vessel carrying mixed blood to the heart, lungs, and systemic circulation. Transportation of the Great Vessels is a condition where vessels or arteries are swapped or they may just be in abnormal positions. Tricuspid Atresia is a condition where there is no tricuspid valve which leads to undersized or absent right ventricle.

Normal heart

Tetralogy of Fallot

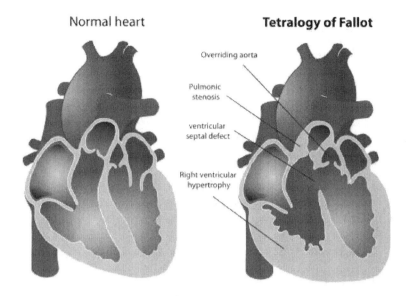

Overriding aorta

Pulmonic
stenosis

ventricular
septal defect

Right ventricular
hypertrophy

Episiotomy- Evaluation of Healing

REEDA

Redness
Edema
Ecchymosis
Discharge, Drainage
Approximation

Redness with pain, excess edema, ecchymosis (bruising), or discharge from the wound can all be signs of problems with healing after an episiotomy. Wound edges should be well approximated. Topical ointments and ice packs may be indicated if there is pain or excess swelling, etc.

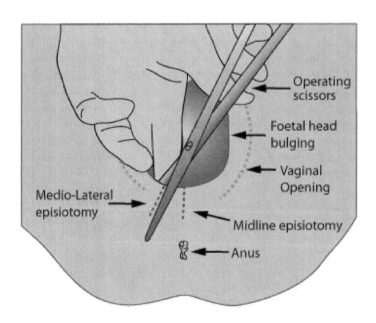

Fetal Accelerations and Decelerations

VEAL CHOP

Variable -	**C**hord Compression
Early -	**H**ead Compression
Accelerations -	**O**kay
Late -	**P**lacental Insufficiency

VEAL CHOP can be used to help remember how to interpret fetal heart rate during labor. For example early decels in FHR(fetal heart rate) indicate head compression. It is typical for decels in FHR during a contraction because of head compression, but FHR should return to normal when contraction ends.

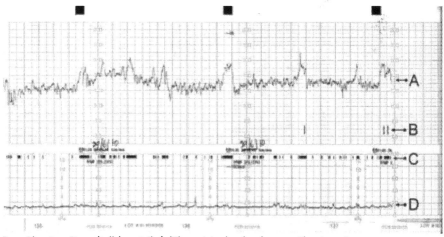

By -- PhantomSteve/talk|contribs\ (The original uploader was Phantomsteve at English Wikipedia) [CC BY-SA 3.0 (http://creativecommons.org/licenses/by-sa/3.0)], via Wikimedia Commons

Fetal Well-Being- Assessment Tests

ALONE

Amniocentesis
L/S Ratio
Oxytocin Test
Non-Stress Test
Estriol Level

An amniocentesis is preformed prenatally. A needle is inserted to obtain a sample of amniotic fluid. The fluid can be used to identify chromosomal abnormalities. L/S ratio compares lecithin–phosphatidyl choline to sphingomyelin to identify infant lung maturity. The oxytocin test measures fetal heart rate during contractions induced by oxytocin. A non-stress test measures fetal heart rate while baby is at rest and while baby is moving. Estriol levels in mother's blood can be a marker for fetal well-being.

Intra Uterine Device- potential problems with use

PAINS

Period (menstrual: late, spotting, bleeding)
Abdominal pain, dyspareunia (painful intercourse)
Infection (abnormal vaginal discharge)
Not feeling well, fever or chills
String missing

An intrauterine device is inserted into the uterus and is used to prevent pregnancy. There are two different types: hormonal and copper IUD.

OB Non-Stress Test -3 negatives in a row to interpret results of Non-Stress Test

NNN

Non-reactive
Non- Stress is
Not good

A non-reactive result in a non-stress is not good. During a non-stress test the fetal heart rate is monitored during movement. A reactive result is a good sign indicating intact central and autonomic nervous system. A reactive non-stress test result would be 2 accelerations to a certain level for greater than 15 seconds within a 20 minute period. If this does not occur the test is non-reactive.

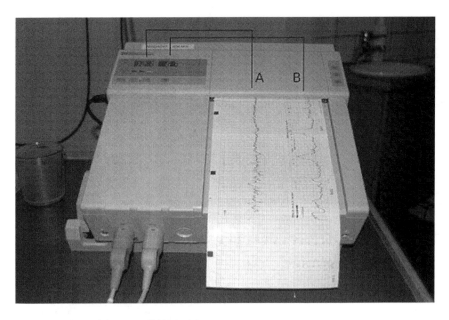

By Steven Fruitsmaak (Own work) [CC BY 3.0
(http://creativecommons.org/licenses/by/3.0)], via Wikimedia Commons

Oral Birth Control Pills- Serious Complications

ACHES

Abdominal Pain
Chest Pain
Headache
Eye Problems
Severe Leg Pain

Monitor for the following serious complications in patients taking oral contraceptives: abdominal pain, chest pain, headache, eye problems, swelling or aching in the legs or thighs.

Post-Partum Assessment

BUBBLE

Breasts
Uterus
Bowels
Bladder
Lochia
Episiotomy-laceration/C-section - incision

Make sure to assess the following in patients postpartum:
1. breasts - engorgement 2. Uterus -check the uterus for bogginess (firming up and dropping to original place 3. Bowel- flatus and bowel movement 4. Bladder – patient will likely have a catheter, check for anything unusual like blood in urine 5. Lochia – discharge 6. Episiotomy-laceration/C-section-incision – check for any signs that wound is not properly healing. (See acronym REEDA to assess episiotomy)

Severe Pre-Eclampsia- Signs and Symptoms

HELLP

Hemolysis
Elevated
Liver function tests
Low
Platelet count

HELLP syndrome is severe high blood-pressure. It typically occurs in the third trimester and usually is found in women that already have a diagnosis of pre-eclampsia. The defining characteristics are hemolysis (breakdown of red blood cells), elevated liver enzymes, and low platelet count.

Hypoxia- Signs and Symptoms (in Pediatrics)

FINES

Feeding difficulty
Inspiratory Stridor
Nares Flares
Expiratory Grunting
Sternal Retractions

The above signs are indications that the patient is attempting to draw in more oxygen. The patient will begin to compensate for the decreased tissue oxygenation by doing the above actions.

Child Abuse/Neglect- Warning Signs

CHILD ABUSE

Childs excessive knowledge on sex and abusive words
Hair growth in various lengths
Inconsistent stories from the child and parent/s
Low self-esteem
Depression

Apathy, no emotion
Bruised
Unusual injuries
Serious injuries
Evidence of old injuries not reported

Child abuse can be in many forms; physical, sexual, emotional, or neglect. Any act of commission or omission by a caregiver that harms or may cause harm to a child is child abuse. As a healthcare professional it is important to be in-tune with the preceding warning signs that can indicate child abuse.

Cleft Lip - Post Op Care

CLEFT LIP

Choking
Lie on back
Evaluate Airway
Feed Slowly
Teaching

Larger nipple opening
Incidence increases in males
Prevent crust formation and aspiration

Cleft lip is a slit in the skin above the lip. Typical treatment is reconstructive surgery. Post op care includes monitoring for choking. Baby will be positioned on back for sleeping to prevent trauma to sutures. Make sure airway is open and monitor for aspiration – baby should be in an upright position for feeding. Feed baby slowly with larger nipple opening. Prevent crust formation. Lastly provide education to parents regarding feeding and common concerns.

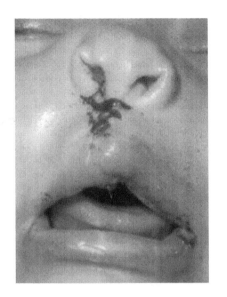

Tracheal Esophageal Fistula- Sign and Symptoms

The 3 Cs

Choking
Coughing
Cyanosis

A congenital abnormality in which there is an opening between the trachea and the esophagus. Surgery is required to repair the opening before a baby can receive po nutrition. Signs and symptoms to identify TEF (tracheal esophageal fistula) are choking, coughing, and cyanosis.

Labs

Hyperkalemia- Causes

The hyperkalemia MACHINE

Medications - ACE Inhibitors, NSAIDS, potassium-sparing diuretics
Acidosis - Metabolic and respiratory
Cellular destruction - burns, traumatic injury, hemolysis
Hypoaldosteronism (Addison's)
Intake- excessive
Nephrons, renal failure
Excretion - Impaired

Hyperkalemia is elevated potassium in the blood. Medications and kidney damage can decrease urinary excretion of potassium. In acidosis and cellular destruction potassium shifts from inside the cell to the blood stream. Excessive intake of potassium can also lead to hyperkalemia. Typical levels of potassium in the blood are 3.7 to 5.2 mEq/L.

Hyperkalemia- Signs and Symptoms

MURDER

Muscle weakness
Urine, oliguria, anuria
Respiratory distress
Decreased cardiac contractility
ECG changes
Reflexes, hyperreflexia, or areflexia (flaccid)

Potassium is necessary for the transmission of electrical impulses in heart and skeletal muscle. Potassium is also a part of reactions that breakdown glucose for energy. It can help maintain acid-base balance.

Hyperkalemia

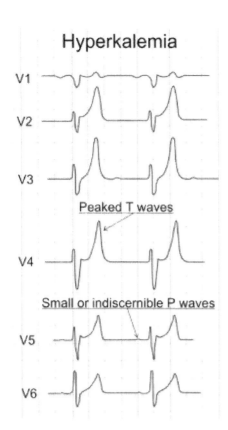

Hyperkalemia- Management

KIND

Kayexalate (orally/ enema)
Insulin
Na HCO3
Diuretics (Furosemide & Thiazides)

The above treatments are utilized to reduce serum potassium levels. Kayexalate works by drawing potassium into the colon. Insulin increases cellular permeability to potassium. Sodium Bicarbonate (NaHCO3) works by increasing blood pH which in turn creates a shift of potassium into the cell as it shifts with the H ion moving out of the cell. Diuretics increase potassium wasting through the urine.

Hypernatremia- Signs and Symptoms

You are FRIED

Fever (low grade), flushed skin
Restless (irritable)
Increased fluid retention and increased BP
Edema (peripheral and pitting)
Decreased urinary output, dry mouth

Hypernatremia is elevated levels of sodium in the blood.
Sodium helps with blood pressure and blood volume. It is also
necessary for muscle and nerve function.

Hypernatremia- Signs and Symptoms

SALT

Skin flushed
Agitation
Low grade fever
Thirst

Hypernatremia is elevated levels of sodium in the blood.
Sodium helps with blood pressure and blood volume. It is also
necessary for muscle and nerve function.

Hypernatremia- Cause

MODEL

Medications /**M**eals

Osmotic diuretics

Diabetes insipidus

Excessive water loss

Low water intake

Hypernatremia is elevated levels of sodium in the blood. It can be caused by excess sodium intake or decrease in free water which leads to a higher concentration of sodium in the blood.

Hypernatremia- Management

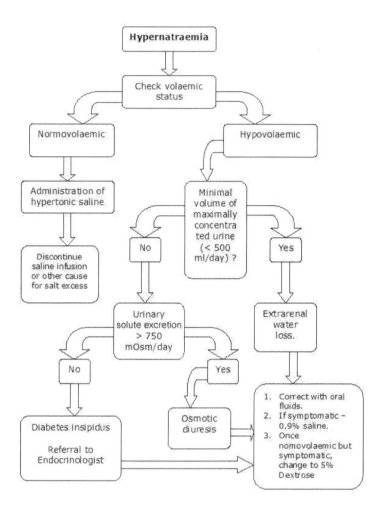

Hypernatremia may either be caused by too much sodium or too little water. First asses volume status of the patient then utilize the chart above to determine best course of action.

Hypocalcemia- Signs and Symptoms

CATS of hypocalcemia

Convulsions
Arrhythmias
Tetany
Spasms and stridor

Hypocalcemia is low levels of Calcium in the blood. Calcium in the blood can be bound to proteins, bound to anions like phosphate, or ionized. Large of stores of Calcium are in bone. Calcium blocks sodium channels, inhibiting depolarization of muscle and nerve fibers. The effects of hypocalcemia are a result of muscle fibers being more excitable

Hyponatremia- Signs and Symptoms

SALT LOSS

Stupor/coma
Anorexia, N&V
Lethargy
Tendon Reflexes decreased

Limp muscles (weakness)
Orthostatic hypotension
Seizures/headache
Stomach cramping

Hyponatremia is decreased levels of sodium in the blood. It can be caused by inadequate sodium or excess free water which leads to lower concentration of sodium.   Sodium and Potassium work together to allow depolarization of muscles. Low sodium levels can limit this ability and cause muscle weakness.
Sodium in the blood helps maintain the oncotic pressure. If fluid leaves the blood vessels that can lead to decreased blood pressure.

Hyponatremia- Signs and Symptoms

SALT LOSS

Stupor/coma
Anorexia, N&V
Lethargy
Tendon Reflexes decreased

Limp muscles (weakness)
Orthostatic hypotension
Seizures/headache
Stomach cramping

Hyponatremia is decreased levels of sodium in the blood. It can be caused by inadequate sodium or excess free water which leads to lower concentration of sodium. Sodium and Potassium work together to allow depolarization of muscles. Low sodium levels can limit this ability and cause muscle weakness.
Sodium in the blood helps maintain the oncotic pressure. If fluid leaves the blood vessels that can lead to decreased blood pressure.

Electrolytes- Location in body

PISO

Potassium
Inside the cell
Sodium
Outside the cell

Potassium and Sodium are the two most abundant cations in the body and have an inverse relationship in regards to intracellular and extracellular concentrations. Potassium is primarily located within the cell and sodium is primarily located outside the cell.

Pharmacology

Beta 1 and Beta 2

Beta 1: heart
Beta 2: lungs
You have one heart and two lungs

Beta 1 adrenergic receptors are mostly found in the heart. Beta 2 adrenergic receptors are found in lungs, GI tract, vascular smooth muscle, skeletal muscle, liver. Beta 1 beta blockers act primarily on the heart. Beta 2 beta blockers act primarily on the lungs.

Drugs for Bradycardia & Low Blood Pressure

IDEA

Isoproterenol
Dopamine
Epinephrine
Atropine Sulfate

We are discussing here SYMPTOMATIC brady and low blood pressure. Bradycardia and hypotension are not necessarily adverse clinical findings in and of themselves.

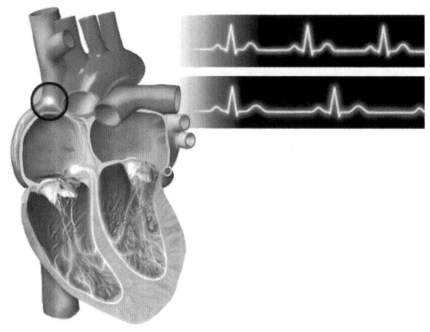

By Blausen Medical Communications, Inc. (Donated via OTRS, see ticket for details) [CC BY 3.0 (http://creativecommons.org/licenses/by/3.0)], via Wikimedia Commons

Drug Interactions

TDCI (These Drugs Can Interact)

Theophylline
Dilantin
Coumadin
Iosone (Erythromycin)

Coumadin and ilosone: ilosone can increase the effects of Coumadin, increase risk for bleeding.
Coumadin and Dilantin: potential for increase effects of both Coumadin and Dilantin
Theophylline and dilantin: if taken orally they can interfere with absorption of each other and decrease medication effect.

Emergency Drugs

Drugs to LEAN on

Lidocaine
Epinephrine
Atropine Sulfate
Narcan

The above drugs work in a variety of emergency settings. Lidocaine can be used in emergency situations for ventricular arrhythmias. Epinephrine is a vital drug in the ACLS protocol. Atropine can be given with symptomatic bradycardia and Narcan is a reversal agent for opiate overdose.

Lidocaine Toxicity

SAMS

Slurred Speech
Altered Central Nervous System
Muscle Twitching
Seizures

Lidocaine is an anesthetic that prevents painful impulses from reaching the brain. In the case of Lidocaine toxicity, look for slurred speech, altered central nervous system, muscle twitching, and seizures.

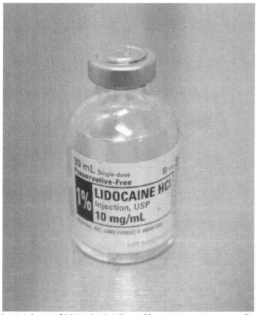

Steroid- Side Effects

6 Ss

Sugar-hyperglycemia
Soggy Bones - causes osteoporosis
Sick - decreased immunity
Sad - depression
Salt - water and salt retention (hypertension)
Sex - decreased libido

Steroids are an effective treatment for asthma, COPD, Crohn's, Lupus and more, however, they carry serious side effects. Steroids can be taken by mouth, via an inhaler, topically, or via injection. Side effects include elevation in blood sugars, elevation in blood pressure (due to water and salt retention), osteoporosis, depression, decreased libido, and decreased immunity.

Mental Health

Anorexia- Signs and Symptoms

ANOREXIA

Amenorrhea delayed
No organic factors accounts for weight loss
Obviously thin but feels FAT
Refusal to maintain normal body weight
Epigastric discomfort is common
X-symptoms (peculiar symptoms)
Intense fears of gaining weight
Always thinking of foods

Anorexia nervosa is an eating disorder characterized by low body weight and periods of starvation, or binging and purging. The lack of adequate nutrition and fat stores can lead to amenorrhea. Patients with anorexia will feel fat even if underweight; anorexia is an unhealthy way to cope with emotional problems. Binging and purging can lead to damage of the GI tract and epigastric discomfort. Some peculiar symptoms may also be seen: abnormal blood counts, bluish discoloration of the fingers, hair that thins, breaks or falls out, or soft downy hair covering the body.

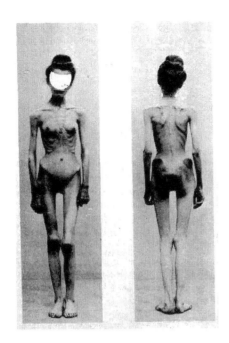

47

Bulimia- Signs and Symptoms

BULIMIA

Binge eating
Under strict dieting
Lacks control/over-eating
Induced vomiting
Minimum of two binge eating episodes
Increase/Persistent concern of body size/shape
Abuse of diuretics and laxatives

Bulimia is an eating disorder characterized by binging and purging. Patients may go through periods of excessive eating and then try to purge be inducing vomiting, taking laxatives or diuretics, or going through periods of fasting.

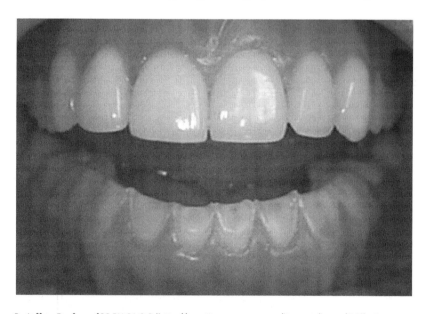

By Jeffrey Dorfman [CC BY-SA 3.0 (http://creativecommons.org/licenses/by-sa/3.0)], via Wikimedia Commons

Bulimia- Signs and Symptoms

WASHED

Weight loss of 15% of original body weight
Amenorrhea
Social withdrawal
History of high activity & achievement
Electrolyte Imbalance
Depression/ Distorted Body Image

Alcoholism- Behavioral Problems

The 5 Ds

Denial
Dependency
Demanding
Destructive
Domineering

Abuse of alcohol can lead to very detrimental outcomes including those listed above. The preceding behavioral problems are common in people suffering from alcoholism.

Alcoholism- Outcome

BAD

Brain Damage
Alcoholic Hallucinations
Death

Abuse of alcohol can lead to very detrimental outcomes including those listed above. Emergent treatment should be provided for patients who have overdosed.

Depression Assessment

SIG

Sleep Disturbances
Interest Decreased
Guilty Feelings

Monitor for these signs and symptoms in patients that may be at risk for depression.

Manic Attack- Signs and Symptoms

DIG FAST

Distractibility
Indiscretion
Grandiosity

Flight of Ideas
Activity Increase
Sleep Deficit
Talkative

The above signs would be indicative of a patient experiencing a manic episode. A manic episode is a state in which the patient experiences abnormally elevated mood.

Alzheimer- Diagnosis

The 5 As

Amnesia – loss of memories
Anomia – unable to recall names of everyday objects
Apraxia – unable to perform tasks of movement
Agnosia – inability to process sensory information
Aphasia – disruption with ability to communicate

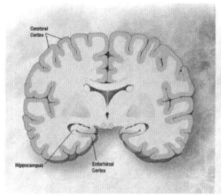 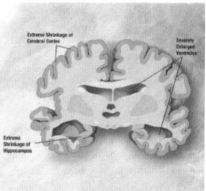

Dementia

DEMENTIA
Make sure they don't have problems with:

Drug and alcohol
Eyes and ears
Metabolic and endocrine disorders
Emotional disorders
Neurologic disorders
Tumors and trauma
Infection
Arteriovascular disease

When assessing a patient for dementia it is important to insure that one of the above listed conditions is an underlying cause for the dementia symptoms.

Senile Dementia- Assess for Changes

JAMCO

Judgment - can a patient determine the outcome of a choice, difficulty assessing risk
Affect - ability to express feeling or emotion
Memory - assess short and long term memory
Cognition- ability to process and relate information
Orientation- assess if a patient is oriented to person, place, time.

Med Surg

Arterial Blood Gases

ROME

Respiratory
Opposite
Metabolic
Equal

	pH	pCO2	HCO3	
Metabolic acidosis	Low	Normal	Low	Equal
Metabolic alkalosis	High	Normal	High	Equal
Respiratory acidosis	Low	High	Normal	Opposite
Respiratory alkalosis	High	Low	Normal	Opposite

First look at the pH: if it is low it is acidosis, high indicates alkalosis. Second use the ROME mnemonic to determine if you have respiratory vs. metabolic.

Pulmonary Edema- Treatment

MAD DOG

Morphine – causes vasodilation resulting in decreased BP
Aminophylline – relaxes airways to make breathing easier
Digitalis – improve heart function in pulmonary edema

Diuretics (Lasix) – pull excess fluid off
Oxygen – improve oxygenation
Gases (Blood Gases ABGs) – asses respiratory status

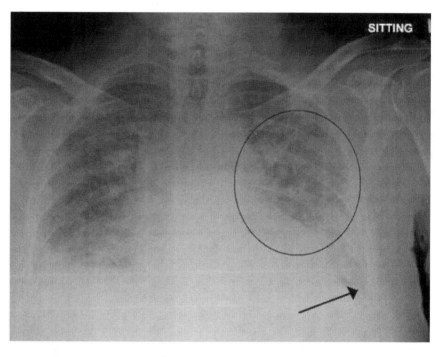

Dyspnea

The 6 Ps

Pulmonary Bronchial Constriction
Possible Foreign Body
Pulmonary Embolus
Pneumothorax
Pump Failure
Pneumonia

Bronchial constriction prevents the passage of air into the lungs which contributes to dyspnea. Foreign bodies can become trapped or logged within the trachea restricting air flow. PE can prevent complete oxygenation of the blood in the alveoli. Pneumothorax collapses the lung and prevents full expansion. Pump failure refers to the heart not beating appropriately. If the heart is not perfusing the lungs than the lungs will be unable to oxygenate the blood. Pneumonia leads to poor lung ventilation as well. These are six major causes for dyspnea.

Hypoxia- Signs and Symptoms

RAT BED

Early Hypoxia:
Restlessness
Anxiety
Tachycardia/ Tachypnea

Late Hypoxia:
Bradycardia
Extreme Restlessness
Dyspnea

Patients experiencing hypoxia will initially demonstrate signs of anxiety and restlessness. As hypoxia continues the patients conditions deteriorates to bradycardia and dyspnea.

Asthma- Management

ASTHMA

Adrenergic (Albuterol)
Steroids
Theophylline
Hydration (IV)
Mask (Oxygen)
Antibiotics

Asthma is a narrowing of the airways. It causes difficulty breathing. Medications can help open the airways.

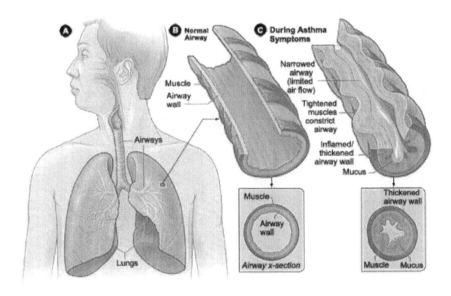

Pupillary reaction

PERRLA

Pupils
Equally
Round and
Reactive to
Light and
Accommodate

Under normal circumstances the pupils will be equally round. The pupils will dilate or constrict in dark or light respectively. The pupils will also accommodate when an item moves closer.

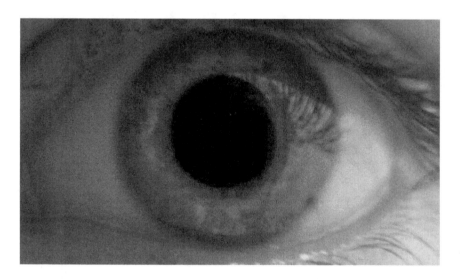

ABCD's

Asymmetry--is the mole irregular in shape?
Border--is the border irregular, notched, or poorly defined?
Color--does the color vary (for example, between shades of brown, red, white, blue, or black)?
Diameter--is the diameter more than 6 mm?

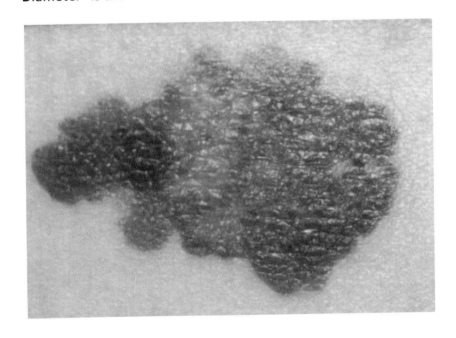

Diabetes Mellitus Type 1 - Signs & Symptoms

The 3 Ps

Polyuria (excessive urination)
Polydypsia (excessive thirst)
Polyphagia (excessive hunger)

In type 1 diabetes mellitus a patient does not produce a hormone called insulin. Insulin allows sugar to go from the blood into the cells for energy. When sugar does not get into the cell sugar levels in the blood rise. The body tries to remove excess glucose by producing extra urine. The body then requires more water. We get hungry because our cells are starving for energy.

Hyperglycemia/Hypoglycemia

Hyper - hot/dry - sugar high
Hypo- cold/clammy - needs candy

During Hyperglycemia a patient is dehydrated, with elevated blood sugars. In hypoglycemia a patient is cold and clammy and need a carbohydrate source to bring their sugars back to a normal range.

Hypoglycemia- Signs and Symptoms

TIRED

Tachycardia
Irritability
Restless
Excessive Hunger
Diaphoresis/ Depression

During hypoglycemia the sugar (glucose) in the blood is too low. Cells of the body can't get adequate energy supply when there is not enough sugar in the blood. You will feel TIRED and have the symptoms listed above.

Circulatory Checks

The 5 Ps

Pain
Paresthesia
Paralysis
Pulse
Pallor (Paleness)

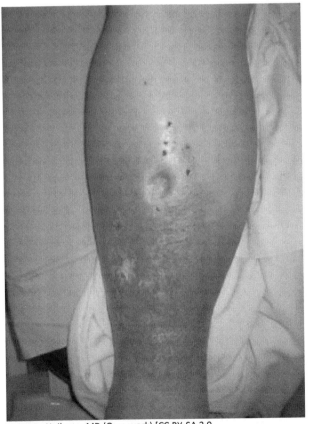

By James Heilman, MD (Own work) [CC BY-SA 3.0
(http://creativecommons.org/licenses/by-sa/3.0) or GFDL
(http://www.gnu.org/copyleft/fdl.html)], via Wikimedia Commons

Hypertension- Nursing Care

DIURETIC

Daily Weight
Intake and Output (I & O)
Urine Output
Response of BP
Electrolytes
Take Pulses
Ischemic Episodes (TIA)
Complications: The 4 Cs on Hypertension (see next page)

For patients with elevated blood pressure monitor daily weights, intake and output, and urine output to watch for fluid retention. Monitor blood pressure and pulse in response to treatments. Diuretics may cause increase loss of electrolytes in the urine.

Hypertension- Complications

The 4 Cs

Coronary Artery Disease
Coronary Rheumatic Fever
Congestive Heart Failure
Cerebral Vascular Accident

Hypertension untreated can lead to vascular and valve destruction including those conditions listed above. Hypertension can also lead CVA or stroke in patients with long term uncontrolled hypertension.

Heart Sounds

APE To Man

Aortic
Pulmonic
Erbs points
Tricuspid
Mitral

This mnemonic is a great reference for cardiac auscultation.

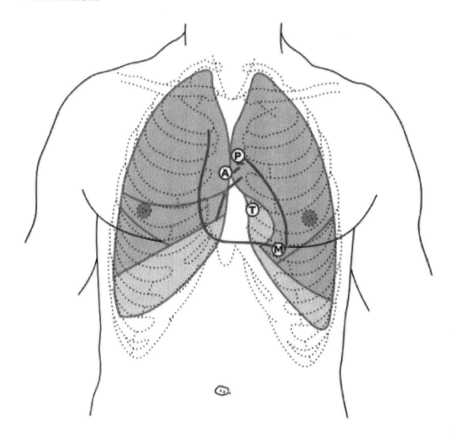

Cardiac Valves Blood Flow

Toilet Paper My A**

Tricuspid
Pulmonic
Mitrial
Aortic

This simple mnemonic helps to remember the order in which blood passes through the four heart valves in sequential order.

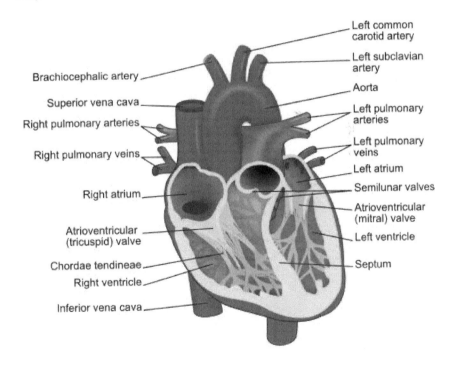

Myocardial Infarction- Immediate Treatment

MONA

Morphine sulfate
Oxygen
Nitroglycerin
ASA (aspirin)

After a myocardial infarction the immediate treatment is morphine sulfate, oxygen, nitroglycerin, and aspirin. Morphine works to decrease pain and difficulty breathing, oxygen insures that poorly oxygenated tissues receive the required O2, nitroglycerin is a potent vasodilator and aids in restoring oxygenation to tissues, aspirin helps to thin the blood and increase tissue perfusion.

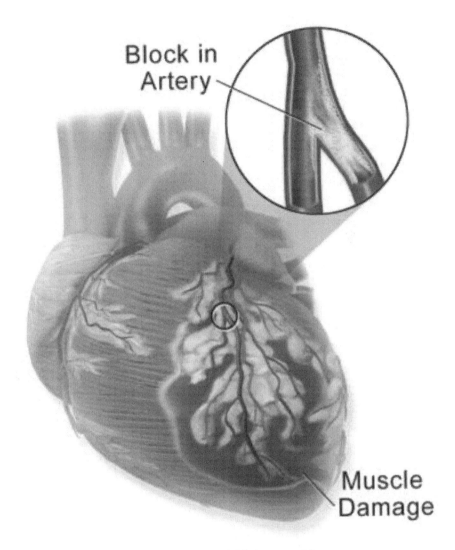

Block in Artery

Muscle Damage

Heart Attack

Myocardial Infarction- Management

MONATAS

Morphine
Oxygen
Nitrates (Nitroglycerin)
Aspirin (ASA)
Thormbolytics
Anti-Coagulants
Stool Softeners

Heart Failure- Right-Sided

HEAD

Hepatomegaly
Edema (Bipedal)
Ascites
Distended Neck Vein

Right sided heart failure will primarily manifest as central edema as the right side of the heart takes fluid from the body and moves it forward. If this portion of the pump is broken fluid will become "backed up" behind the pump . . . within the body.

Heart Failure- Left-Sided

CHOP

Cough
Hemoptysis
Orthopnea
Pulmonary Congestion (crackles/ rales)

Left sided heart failure will primarily manifest as pulmonary edema as the left side of the heart moves blood from the lungs throughout the body. If this portion of the pump is broken the blood will become "backed up" within the lungs. Left sided heart failure can often lead to right sided heart failure.

CHF- Treatment

UNLOAD FAST

U sit Upright
Nitro
Lasix
Oxygen
Aminophylline
Digoxin

Fluids - decrease
Afterload - decrease
Sodium - decrease
Tests: dig level, ABG, K+

These treatments used in conjunction will help in reducing the symptoms and complications associated with CHF.

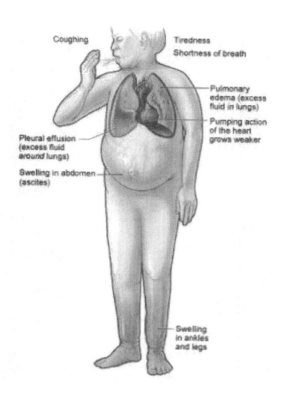

Coughing

Tiredness

Shortness of breath

Pulmonary edema (excess fluid in lungs)

Pumping action of the heart grows weaker

Pleural effusion (excess fluid around lungs)

Swelling in abdomen (ascites)

Swelling in ankles and legs

Inflammation- Signs and Symptoms

HIPER

Heat
Indurations (hardening)
Pain
Edema
Redness

In response to tissue damage the body elicits the inflammatory response in attempt to rid itself of the initial offender. These attempts can sometimes become more of a problem than a help.

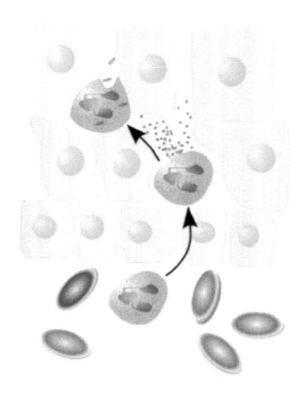

Toxicty/Sepsis- Signs and Symptoms

The 6 T's:

Tachycardia
Tachypnea
Tremors
Toxic look
Tiredness
Temperature (fever)

Sepsis is a systemic response to inflammation as a result of uncontrolled infection there is also a release of cytokines which lead to further inflammation and vascular dilation. Blood is shunted from the essential organs to non essential organs (the skin) leading to increased body temperature (along with response to infection). The heart begins to beat faster in response to the infection and to the decreased cardiac output as a result of the massive vasodilation.

Cancer- Early Warning Signs

CAUTION UP

Change in bowel or bladder
A lesion that does not heal
Unusual bleeding or discharge
Thickening or lump in breast or elsewhere
Indigestion or difficulty swallowing
Obvious changes in wart or mole
Nagging cough or persistent hoarseness

Unexplained weight loss
Pernicious Anemia

Cancer can sometimes be difficult to identify, but the earlier it is detected the better chance treatment will be effective.

Cancer- Interventions

CANCER

Comfort
Altered Body Image
Nutrition
Chemotherapy
Evaluate response to meds
Respite for caretakers

Leukemia- Signs and Symptoms

ANT

Anemia
Neutropenia
Thrombocytopenia

Leukemia can lead to anemia as it will disrupt the production of blood within the bone marrow. Neutropenia is a natural result of leukemia as the bodies supply of white blood cells is decreased. Thrombocytopenia is a reduced platelet count which can result from leukemia especially in infants.

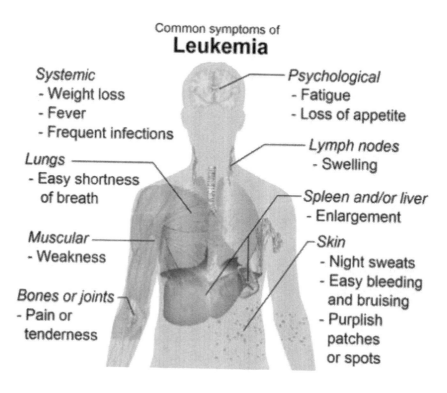

Common symptoms of
Leukemia

Systemic
- Weight loss
- Fever
- Frequent infections

Lungs
- Easy shortness
  of breath

Muscular
- Weakness

Bones or joints
- Pain or
  tenderness

Psychological
- Fatigue
- Loss of appetite

Lymph nodes
- Swelling

Spleen and/or liver
- Enlargement

Skin
- Night sweats
- Easy bleeding
  and bruising
- Purplish
  patches
  or spots

Appendicitis- Assessment

PAINS

Pain (RLQ) - pain in the right lower quadrant of the abdomen
Anorexia - loss of appetite
Increased temperature, WBC (15,000-20,000)
Nausea
Signs (McBurney's, Psoas)

> <u>Psoas</u> sign is pain when a patient extends their thigh while lying on their side with knees extended. It indicates irritation to certain muscles in the abdomen.
>
> <u>McBurney's</u> sign is if there is deep tenderness at mcBurney's point - right side of the abdomen, one-third the distance from the anterior superior iliac spine to the navel

Epiglottitis - Signs and Symptoms

AIR RAID

Airway Closed
Increased Pulse
Restlessness

Retractions- occur when the muscles between the ribs pull inward
Anxiety Increased
Inspiratory Stridor- high-pitched breath sound resulting from turbulent air flow in the larynx
Drooling

> The epiglottis is a flap of cartilage that covers the entrance to our airway when we swallow food. Inflammation of the epiglottis can close of the airway.

Cholinergic Crisis

SLUD

Salivation
Lacrimation
Urination
Defecation

A cholinergic crisis can occur if the body stops properly breaking down acetlycholine. This can cause an overstimulation of the neuromuscular junction.

Adrenal Gland Hormones

The 3 Ss

Sugar (Glucocorticoids)
Salt (Mineralcorticoids)
Sex (Androgens)

There are three different adrenal gland hormones which can be remembered as the 3 Ss: sugar (Glucocorticoids) effect glucose utilization, fat metabolism and aid in reducing inflammation, salt (Mineralcorticoids) play a role in electrolyte regulation, sex (Androgens) commonly referred to as sex hormones.

Cranial Nerve Mnemonic 01

Olympic Opium Occupies Troubled Triathletes After
Finishing Vegas Gambling Vacations Still High

Olfactory
Optic
Oculomotor
Trochlear
Trigeminal
Abducens
Facial
Vestibulocochlear
Glossopharyngeal
Vagus
Spinal Accessory
Hypoglossal

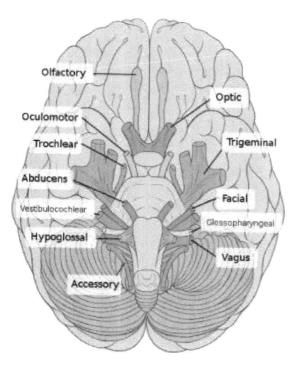

Cranial Nerve Mnemonic 02

Oh Oh Oh To Touch And Feel Very Good Velvet AH!

Olfactory
Optic
Oculomotor
Trochlear
Trigeminal
Abducens
Facial
Vestibulocochlear
Glossopharyngeal
Vagus
Accessory
Hypoglossal

Cranial Nerve Mnemonic 03

On Old Obando Tower Top A Filipino Army Guards Villages
And Huts

Olfactory
Optic
Oculomotor
Trochlear
Trigeminal
Abducens
Facial
Vestibulocochlear
Glossopharyngeal
Vagus
Accessory
Hypoglossal

Cranial Nerve Mnemonics- Sensory, Motor or Both

1: Some Say Marilyn Monroe But My Brother Says Bridget Bardot Mmm Mmm

2: Some Say Marry Money But My Brother Says Bad Business Marry Money

Olfactory	Sensory
Optic	Sensory
Oculomotor	Motor
Trochlear	Motor
Trigeminal	Both
Abducens	Motor
Facial	Both
Vestibulocochlear	Sensory
Glossopharyngeal	Both
Vagus	Both
Accessory	Motor
Hypoglossal	Motor

Prostate

Prostate Problems are no... FUN

Frequency
Urgency
Nocturia

As a patient begins to develop prostate issues they will start to demonstrate urinary symptoms including those listed above.

Diarrhea- treatment

Banana
Rice
Apple
Toast

The BRAT diet is a bland diet that is low in protein, fiber, and fat. It is thought to be easy on the GI tract and helpful to lesson diarrhea. It is not used commonly any more because of the lack of protein in the diet.

Transient Incontinence- Common Causes

DIAPPERS

Delirium
Infection
Atrophic Urethra- atrophy of the urethra
Pharmaceuticals- blood pressure medication,
antidepressants, diuretics, sleeping pills
Psychologic
Excess Urine Output
Restricted Mobility
Stool Impaction

Promotion and Evaluation of Normal Elimination

POOPER SCOOP

(Promotion)
Position
Output
Offer Fluids
Privacy
Exercise
Report Results

(Evaluation)
Size (Amount)
Consistency
Occult Blood
Odor
Peristalsis

Bleeding Precautions

RANDI

Razor Electric/ Blades
Aspirin
Needles- small gauge
Decrease needle sticks
Injury (Protect from)

If a patient is taking an anticoagulant to prevent blood clots there is increase risk for bleeding. Be careful with blades when shaving. Do not take aspirin as it interferes with blood clotting and can magnify the effect of your medication. Avoid excess needle sticks and protect the patient from injury.

Trauma- Complications

TRAUMATIC

Tissue Perfusion Problems
Respiratory Problems
Anxiety
Unstable Clotting Factors
Malnutrition
Altered Body Image
Thromboembolism- fat embolism
Infection
Coping Problems

In trauma the patient needs to be quickly assessed for adequate perfusion as part of the trauma survey. Trauma can lead to overt or covert blood loss resulting in shock. If there is significant blood loss the patient may develop disseminated intravascular coagulation as they begin to deplete their available clotting factors.

Trauma- Assessment (Emergency)

ABCDEFGHI

Airway
Breathing
Circulation
Disability
Examine
Fahrenheit
Get Vitals
Head to Toe Assessment
Intervention

Rapid assessment and treatment of the trauma patient is essential to their overall survival. Working through this framework will aid in remembering where to focus your efforts. Always remember your ABC and patient safety. Once those things have been secured you can move on to less vital components.

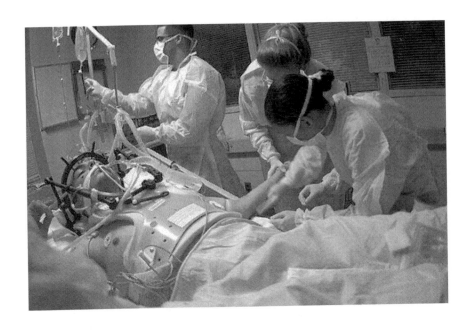

Trauma Surgery- After initial assessment

AMPLE

Allergies
Medications
Past Medical History
Last Meal
Events Surrounding Injury

Exercise Guidelines

FIT

Frequency (3x per week)
Intensity (60-80% of Maximal Heart Rate)
Time (Aerobic Activity)

Osteoporosis- Risk Factors

ACCESS

Alcohol Use
Corticosteroid Use
Calcium low
Estrogen low
Smoking
Sedentary lifestyle/s

ACCESS leads to OSTEOPOROSIS

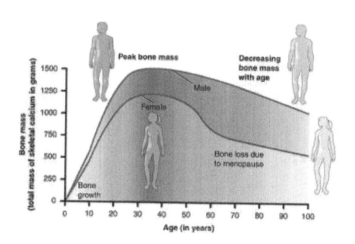

By Anatomy & Physiology, Connexions Web site. http://cnx.org/content/col11496/1.6/, Jun 19, 2013. (OpenStax College) [CC BY 3.0 (http://creativecommons.org/licenses/by/3.0)], via Wikimedia Commons

Dialysis- Who needs dialysis?

Check the vowels: AEIOU

Acid-Base Problems
Electrolyte Problems
Intoxications
Overload of fluids
Uremic Symptoms

As a patient progresses from chronic kidney disease to end stage renal disease the need for dialysis becomes more imminent. When the kidneys are no longer able to filter the blood alone you will see problem metabolic acidosis since they kidneys can't excrete excess acids that are in the blood. During kidney failure excess potassium isn't excreted and levels will start to rise. The kidneys help remove certain medications from the body, and when they aren't working toxicity can occur even with normal doses. Patients with ESRD become fluid overloaded due to inadequate urine production. Uremia will occur as the body can't excrete enough urea.

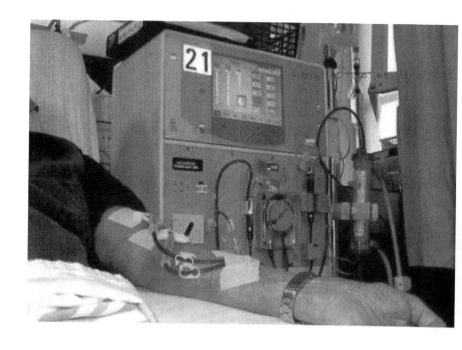

Gluten Free Diet

BROW

Barley
Rye
Oats
Wheat

Gluten is a protein found in wheat, barley and rye. People with gluten allergies can be affected by even trace amount of gluten in foods. Oats do not contain gluten, but they are often milled in the same factories as wheat. Always check food labels to make sure a product is gluten free

Nursing Fundamentals

Body Systems

MR DICE RUNS

Muscle
Respiratory

Digestive
Integumentary
Circulatory
Endocrine

Reproductive
Urinary
Nervous
Skeletal

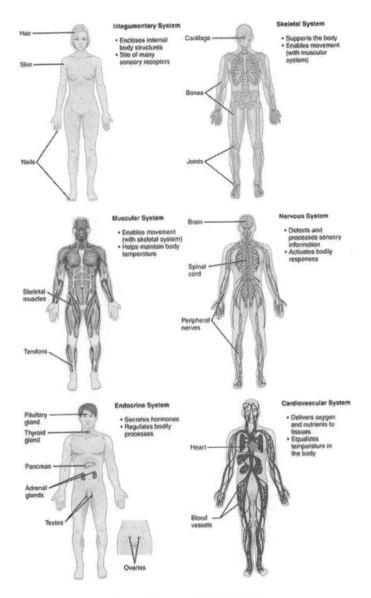

Steps in the Nursing Process

ADPIE (A Delicious PIE)

Assessment
Diagnosis
Planning
Implementation
Evaluation

Steps in the Nursing Process

AAPIE (An Apple PIE)

Assessment
Analysis
Planning
Implementation
Evaluation

Sprains and Strains- Nursing Care

RICE

Rest
Ice
Compression
Elevation

Traction- Nursing Care

TRACTION

Temperature (Extremity, Infection)
Ropes hang freely
Alignment
Circulation Check (5 Ps)
Type & Location of fracture
Increase fluid intake
Overhead trapeze
No weights on bed or floor

ADLs (Activity of Daily Living)

BATTED

Bathing
Ambulation
Toileting
Transfers
Eating
Dressing

When assessing a patient's ability to care for themself at home we must assess their ability to complete activities of daily living. A patient's ability to bath, walk, and toilet on their own will help us determine the level of care they will need when they leave the hospital.

IADLS (Instrumental Activities of Daily Living)

SCUM

Shopping
Cooking and Cleaning
Using telephone or transportation
Managing money and medications

The instrumental activities of daily living are used to determine a patient's ability to carry out necessary functions for independent living. If they are unable to manage the activities above, they will likely require some sort of assistance from family or a home health agency, etc.

Canes

COAL

Cane
Opposite
Affected
Leg

When teaching a patient how to walk with a cane it is important to instruct them to keep the cane on the opposite side of the affected extremity.

Walkers

Wandering Wilmas Always Late

Walker
With
Affected
Leg

When walking with a walker the patient should lift the walker as they lift their affected leg. This allows for the "good" leg to support the movement of the walker.

About the Authors

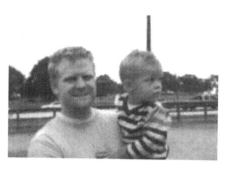

Sick of spending hours and hours trying to find all the information you need for clinical and NCLEX® study? So was I . . . . That's why I created NRSNG.com, a community of nurses and nursing students wanting to jump start their careers.

I am a registered nurse and CCRN on a Neurovascular Intensive Care Unit at a Level I Trauma Hospital. I attended college at Brigham Young University and later received my Nursing degree from Methodist College in Peoria, IL. I also hold a Business Management degree from Touro University.

Professionally, I precept nursing students and new graduate Registered Nurses and work as a charge nurse . . . and love it!

Come visit us at NRSNG.com or check in on Facebook.com/NRSNG.

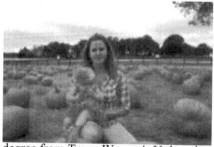

Sandra is a dietitian with one of the largest health care systems in the United States. She works with intensive care patients. She obtained her undergraduate degree from Brigham Young University and her graduate degree from Texas Woman's University. She holds advanced certifications in nutrition support management.

Reviews greatly help this book reach more students. Click below to leave a review on Amazon or to share the book on Facebook. Nothing helps more than a few kind words.

Your Free Gift!

As a way of saying thanks for your purchase, I'm offering a free PDF download:

"63 Must Know NCLEX® Labs"

With these charts you will be able to take the 63 most important labs with you anywhere you go!

You can download the 4 page PDF document by clicking here, or going to NRSNG.com/labs

Made in the USA
Lexington, KY
18 December 2015